Sleeping wit

By Dr Sue Peacock

ISBN-13: 978-0-9954599-2-2

Published by Ann Jaloba Publishing, 26 Tapton Mount Close, Sheffield S10 5DJ

Note to Readers

DEDICATION

I would like to thank my family, particularly my husband Steve, who now knows far more about chronic pain and sleep than he ever wished to know! I thank them all for their love, support and encouragement.

All of the people living with chronic pain who participated in my programmes and the MK Chronic Pain Support Group who regularly hears about my new projects, I thank them for giving me their time so freely, giving their honest opinions, supporting my new projects and sharing with me their experiences of living with chronic pain.

Finally, I would like to thank my dear friend and mentor Dr Jane Porter, who has always willingly shared her valuable knowledge and insight, teaching me so much about chronic pain over the years.

sleeping with pain

Contents

sleeping with pain

ABOUT SUE

Dr Sue Peacock is a Consultant Health Psychologist and Head of The Health Psychology Service at Milton Keynes Hospital NHS Foundation Trust. She is registered with the Health and Care Professions Council and is an Associate Fellow of The British Psychological Society. She has a PhD in pain psychology.
Sue is also an Advanced Hypnotherapy Practitioner registered on the General Hypnotherapy Register, an EMDR practitioner and has diplomas in neuro-linguistic programming and life coaching.

In addition to this, she has her own thriving private practice, providing specialist psychological therapy to clients and various training programmes to health professionals. The focus is on improving people's ability to manage their health conditions and adjust to the different circumstances and challenges faced. With her help, Sue's clients find that stress reduces and the quality of their general life can improve. The ultimate aim is to enable clients to live fulfilling lives despite their health conditions.

Sue is active in research. Her research interests include sleep and pain; ethnic and cultural differences in perceptions of pain, and the impact on how people experience living with long term pain and other long-term health conditions. Current research is looking at the role of emotional contagion within a pain management programme and how social media and technology can be used to help young people to adhere to treatment plans.

She has been involved in teaching health professionals about psychological aspects of pain at Masters Level, and regularly holds study days in the areas of pain management and health psychology. Additionally she supervises trainee health psychologists on placement offering opportunities in Consultancy and Psychological Interventions.

FOREWORD

"Pete, would you write the foreword for my book I'm writing about pain and sleep," asked Sue.

She didn't have to ask me twice, because after 20 plus years of self-managing my pain, getting a decent night's sleep is a challenge.

I would say around 90 percent of the people with pain who contact me via the Pain Toolkit website (www.paintoolkit.org) say one of their main problems is sleep. I'm guessing as you're reading Sue's book, you are one of the 90 percent, so you're not on your own.

So what about Sue's book? I have to be honest I'm not one of those guys who learns from reading. I'm more of visual learner.

But I have to say this book grabbed my attention. It provided with very simple information about sleep, I hadn't heard or read before.

What I really liked about it was the little simple exercises in it, which made me think. The text wasn't like other books telling me what to do, but it was giving me what they call food for thought. It's interactive.

I really liked the 'Over to you sections.' Check these bits out. They are really good.

I also liked the section where it talked about setting goals. This is really important for people with pain. Because each day usually melts into the next one, setting goals or smaller ones called action plans isn't something we do.

Lastly, this is a book that encourages the reader to say to themselves: "I think I can do this."

I've tried out some of the techniques and I'm pleased to say . . . YES! YES! YES! I've had quite a few nights where I've slept better. But it's like everything in pain management, we need to keep practising and of course keep it up.

Good luck with your newly found sleep friend called *Sleeping with Pain*.

Pete Moore
Author of Pain Toolkit and Pain Tips

INTRODUCTION

Sleep is a built-in ability that usually doesn't take much effort at all. I mean, how simple can it be to sleep? You just close your eyes, relax and get taken away to your dreams. However for many, many people, sleeping isn't as easy as that.

I once asked one of my chronic pain patients what does insomnia mean to you? Her reply was 1.51 am + eternity + 1.52 am + eternity + 1.53 am + eternity!

Perhaps this is you. It's dark, it's nearly 2 am, and you still haven't slept despite going to bed at 1. You toss and turn, count sheep, pull the bedcovers up, then throw them off, you look at the clock again. Its only five minutes since you last looked but it feels like forever! It feels terrible and you do not know what to do next.

sleeping with pain

Your pain is getting worse and you have taken all your allocated medication, you're tempted to take extra, but you would have to get up and it's cold so you continue lying there, feeling frustrated and getting more and more wound up because you can't sleep. Everyone in your house is asleep, your partner's snoring is echoing through the whole house. Eventually, you nudge your beloved gently, then nudge a bit harder. Because you really want them to wake up and chat, because everyone in the whole world is sleeping except you!

If this is familiar, read on!

According to a 2011 report by the Mental Health Foundation, a third of the UK's population suffers from insomnia severe enough to affect their health. The Chief Medical Officer's report in 2008 says 86 percent of people with chronic pain reported an inability to sleep well.

Famous author, F. Scott Fitzgerald once wrote, "The worst thing in the world is to try to sleep and not to." He was not exaggerating, Sleep is meant to revive us and get us ready to 'live for another day'. When people are denied sleep, the effects can be devastating.

It is known that insomnia, pain and psychological distress are intertwined; therefore a combination approach works best. It is possible to overcome insomnia. It's not easy, but it can be done and this book will show you how. This is how it works.

In this book, I'll explore what sleep is and what causes insomnia. I also look in depth at the insomnia which comes when people are in chronic pain. I will help you change your thoughts, bedtime rituals, environment and re-programme your sleep so you finally get a good night's sleep! In order to get the most out of this book, I would suggest that you get a notebook or journal so you can answer the questions posed throughout this book, in the 'over to you' sections and you can record important information about your sleep.

Also set time aside in your day to concentrate on the tasks I suggest throughout the book. Don't pick and choose the tasks you like best or find easiest. For the greatest effect on the quality of your sleep you need to do them all! Doing these things will give you the maximum chance of improving your quality of sleep.

You can find out more about my work with chronic pain at www.apaininthemind.co.uk and download complimentary downloads including fact sheets, top tips and audios, suitable for people with pain or health professionals working with people with chronic pain. On this website you will find a range of programmes and information on how you can book your own bespoke pain management programme and/or sleeping with pain programme with me.

Dr Sue Peacock

sleeping with pain

Chapter 1:

HOW DOES PAIN AFFECT SLEEP?

Chronic pain and insomnia appear to go hand in hand, with the vast majority of chronic pain patients reporting disturbed, interrupted or poor quality of sleep. Nearly eight million people in UK have chronic pain, and two thirds of these report sleep problems. That's millions of people in misery every day.

For people experiencing chronic pain, a doctor will often make a diagnosis of 'secondary insomnia', that is, sleep problems directly attributable to the pain. However, due to the complex nature of chronic pain many people experience emotional issues as well. And if that wasn't enough, it is common for sleep to be affected by prescribed pain medications.

Disrupted sleep will, in turn, increase the chronic pain problem. Therefore, this becomes a vicious cycle in which the pain disrupts your sleep, and difficulty sleeping makes your pain worse, which in turn makes sleeping more difficult and so the cycle continues.

Chronic pain can disrupt your sleep in many ways. Often the best way to understand how chronic pain can make it difficult to fall asleep is to think about the process associated with going to sleep at night. While getting ready for bed, we often try to eliminate all distractions or influences, by turning off the lights, trying to get comfortable in an effort to try to 'relax' and begin to fall asleep.

Pain increases as you try to sleep

However, these activities which make our environment quieter can cause problems if we suffer with chronic pain, because the only thing left to focus on *is* the experience of pain. Many of my patients report that one of their main pain management strategies during the day is distracting themselves from their pain by being involved in various activities and staying busy.

When it comes to trying to fall asleep, there are no other distractions to focus upon. There is just their perception of their pain. Often, the perception of pain actually *increases* when trying to go to sleep. The longer it takes to fall asleep, the more stressful the situation becomes and the more pain is experienced, so the vicious cycle continues.

In addition to the difficulty of actually getting to sleep, many people with chronic pain report waking up frequently throughout the night.

People experiencing chronic pain may experience several 'micro-arousals' every hour of sleep which lead to awakenings. These micro-arousals are a change of the sleep state to a lighter stage of sleep. So chronic pain can be a significant intrusion into the night's sleep and very disruptive to the normal stages of sleep.

This is often the cause of 'non-restorative sleep' where the person with chronic pain still feels tired and unrefreshed even though they have slept during the night.

People with chronic pain often experience less deep sleep, more arousals and awakenings during the night as well as less efficient sleep. This non-restorative sleep can then lead to lack of energy, low mood, fatigue and increased pain during the day. We are now beginning to understand more about these processes and this means we can get some control. But before we go on to that we are going to look at what pain is, what it does and what happens when it starts sending our brains the wrong messages. So, if you want to understand more about pain go on to the next chapter.

sleeping with pain

Chapter 2:

UNDERSTANDING YOUR PAIN

Everyone knows that pain is a universal human experience and something we all suffer from at some time in our lives. However, there are different types of pain and sometimes the pain signals our brains are processing are not working for our good.

Chronic pain, in particular has its own characteristics. So if we want to understand pain better a good place to start is by looking at the difference between chronic pain and the short term pain most of us will experience at one time or another. There is constant research going on into pain and we are coming to understand this complex condition better all the time. What we do know from current research is that the experience of pain depends on how our brain processes experiences. This is true of both chronic and acute pain.

Acute pain: a warning signal

If you have had pain for a defined amount of time, whether that is a few days or weeks, this is called acute pain. It is often associated with tissue damage such as a back injury or sprained ankle. Pain is unpleasant and in the case of acute pain it does an important job as it acts as a warning signal that something is wrong with the workings of our bodies.

Pain demands our attention and interrupts our usual activities, thoughts and emotions. We want answers or an explanation about our pain and pain insists that we get help to relieve it. Our brains interpret this as a 'threat response' and whilst our brains receive these signals it will behave as if we are in danger. In this situation, our brains release chemicals which cause us to take appropriate action to protect our damaged bodies.

Our muscles become tense and more protective chemicals are released in the body to guard against more damage. Thoughts such as worry and anxiety appear to do a job, they create chemicals which are released to try and help us find out what is wrong and why we have pain.

The stress of having pain causes further chemicals to be released into our bodies to try and make us respond and get help. Our whole system is on a high alert as everything works to protect us and put the damage right.

Depending upon the type of injury, acute pain is normally relieved either by time as the natural healing process kicks in, hands on physiotherapy, some form of medical or surgical treatment, pain killers, or a mixture of all or some of the above. Sometimes it can be relieved without medical treatments. The general advice is stay active and gradually return to your everyday activities such as work, social life and gentle exercise.

Chronic pain: your over-active system

If you have had pain for three months or more, then it is classified as chronic or persistent pain. This type of pain is common and can be caused by conditions such as arthritis or nerve damage or a result of an injury or problem that has often healed but left a residual problem. Sometimes it develops slowly over time as result of an injury or surgery; sometimes it develops for no identifiable reason.

Chronic pain is different to acute pain as it doesn't go away and often doesn't respond to treatments, even where many different things are tried.

After three to six months, the body has usually healed as well as can be expected. So what is going on if you are still in pain?

The answer lies in the nervous system. The on-going pain that is still being produced is less about the injuries within the body and more about the sensitivity of the nervous system. This makes it more complex to treat but if we understand what is happening we can make some effective interventions. So why do our nervous systems behave like this? Chronic pain is triggered when the nerves carrying unpleasant and unhelpful information become irritated and continue to react even when the issue which caused the pain in the first place has healed. It's as if the pain system stays switched on.

A good way to understand this is to use the analogy of of a burglar alarm. Lights flash and loud sounds are emitted from the alarm when someone is trying to break into your house. This grabs your attention so you can react to it and a good thing too. However alarms are frustrating, irritating and annoying when they go off for the wrong reasons, say because a spider or fly goes into the sensor. The loud noise is still emitted, the lights flash but no-one is breaking into your house and there is no danger. The noise is just annoying and disruptive.

We can apply this analogy to chronic pain. In chronic pain, the pain sensing nerves are sending off the same 'threat' chemicals as if there was an instant threat of danger or injury when none exists and this pattern keeps repeating itself. Your nervous system notices anything that might make it react, such as lack of sleep, over-activity, under-activity, the weather, your mood and stress levels.

What you can do to alleviate chronic pain

Once a chronic pain problem has been thoroughly and completely investigated and treated – without success – it may have to be accepted that there is no known cure at present.

That doesn't mean you just have to accept the pain. There are things you can do. The very best way to tackle chronic pain is to learn how we can affect our pain system ourselves, by what we do, by what we think and by learning how to really relax.

It helps to consider chronic pain from a broad perspective and look at all aspects of your life. So many things could potentially affect your nervous system and may be contributing to your pain experience.

Keeping active is very important as it sends the right signals to your brain.

Never under-estimate the importance of keeping active. This is best achieved through pacing and goal setting, which if used appropriately will reduce the chance of a 'flare up' of your pain. Your brain needs to see you getting moving without fear at levels where your pain is manageable. When your brain begins to register this is will stop trying to protect you from the pain.

Consider your thoughts and feelings about your pain and how they affect your nervous system. Living with chronic pain impacts on all aspects of your life and this affects your mood and stress levels. Remember all those thoughts and feelings are brain impulses too which can lead to the 'threat' chemicals being released. It is important to learn to manage your thoughts, feelings and your stress, so you can turn down the signals within the nervous system. This will help with your sleep, emotional wellbeing and can ease pain.

Deeper meanings

Many people with pain find exploring the deeper meaning of pain and their personal story surrounding their pain can be extremely beneficial. Try to look back at everything that was happening in your life around the time your pain started. Often you will be able to recognise useful links between a worrying period of life and increasing worry about their pain, which can be part of the healing process.

So in summary, if you have chronic pain try to
- exercise,
- stay fairly relaxed
- pace your activity

If you do this, you will be likely to experience less pain, and therefore sleep more easily. The person with chronic pain who does not keep fit, and who does nothing to keep busy, is prone to being tense and, will be likely to experience more pain and find it more difficult to sleep.

You have a measure of control. This means that what you do can affect the amount of pain you experience at any one time. You can make it better or worse. So look at the questions and spend some time answering them to gain an insight into your unique experience. Then we will look at the mystery of sleep in more detail in the next chapter.

Over to you - Understanding your Pain

Understanding your pain is

important and will help you cope

better with it. In your notebook

or journal answer the following

questions:

1.   What is acute pain?

2.   What is chronic pain?

3.   What may cause chronic pain?

4.   What activities may help you manage your pain

      more effectively?

5.   What exercise do I do, or could I do?

6.   Are there any links between the onset of my pain

      and a difficult time in my life?

Summarise your understanding of pain in 2-3 sentences

maximum.

sleeping with pain

Chapter 3:

UNDERSTANDING THE SLEEP CYCLE

We don't think about sleep until it becomes a problem for us! Sleep isn't a luxury, sufficient and restful sleep is a human need as basic as food, vital to emotional and physical well-being. In recent years, scientists have made great strides in identifying patterns and functions of brain activity in sleep.

Sleep is commonly misunderstood; it is not simply the absence of wakefulness; it is much more complex than that. Sleep varies across the night and for most of us throughout the night as well. Sleep varies with age and stages of development. Most importantly sleep varies from person to person! It is an active process with physical, mental and emotional components.

We need sleep from a physical perspective as it restores and recuperates our tissues, it allows time for our tired muscles to recover. At a deeper level within the body, new proteins are synthesised and hormones are produced.

Sleep loss affects our mental health as it causes inattention, memory problems, fatigue, drowsiness, inability to stay awake and disorientation, and that's without your strong painkillers!

Lack of sleep also affects our emotional health; our physical well-being depends upon sleep. We have all experienced irritability through lack of sleep, it can also make us feel over-anxious or over-excited and our mood may become downbeat.

The circadian rhythms

Sleep is a process made up of different types and subtypes which are organised in a series of cycles repeated through the night.

The daily cycle of life, which includes sleeping and waking, is called a *circadian* (meaning 'about a day') rhythm, commonly referred to as the biological clock. Hundreds of bodily functions follow biological clocks, but sleeping and waking are the most important circadian rhythms.

Light signals coming through the eyes reset the circadian cycles each day. The response to light signals in the brain is an important key factor in sleep and in maintaining a normal circadian rhythm. Light signals travel to a tiny cluster of nerves in the hypothalamus in the centre of the brain, the body's master clock, which is called the *supra chiasmatic nucleus* or SCN. This nerve cluster takes its name from its location, which is just above (*supra*) the optic chiasm. The optic chiasm is a major junction for nerves transmitting information about light from the eyes.

The approach of dusk each day prompts the *supra chiasmatic nucleus* (SCN) to signal the nearby *pineal gland* (named so because it resembles a pine-cone) to produce the hormone melatonin. Melatonin is an important hormone released in the brain that may be critical for the body's time-setting. The longer a person is in darkness the longer melatonin is secreted. Levels drop after staying in bright light. Research is ongoing to determine if high levels of melatonin cause sleep regardless of whether it is dark.

The sleep-wake cycles in humans are designed to produce activity during the day and sleep at night. There is also is a natural peak in sleepiness at mid-day, the traditional siesta time. The sleeping and waking cycle is approximately 24 hours. If confined to windowless apartments, with no clocks or other time cues, sleeping and waking as their bodies dictate, humans typically live on slightly longer than 24-hour cycles.

In sleep studies, subjects spend about one-third of their time asleep, suggesting that most people need about eight hours of sleep each day. Infants may sleep as many as 16 hours a day. Older adults may sleep less at night, approximately six to six and a half hours per night, but have a tendency to 'top up' with naps in the daytime. Individual adults differ in the amount of sleep they need to feel well rested, so this is something worth remembering if you don't seem to fit the average. Daily rhythms intermesh with a number of biological and physical factors that may interfere or change individual patterns. For example, the firing of nerve cells in the brain may be faster or slower in different individuals. Such differences are fractions of a second but they can cause variations in the type, timing, and duration of a person's sleep.

The importance of sunlight as a cue for circadian rhythms is shown very clearly by the problems experienced by people who are totally blind: they commonly suffer trouble sleeping and other rhythm disruptions.

The different states of sleep

Sleep consists of two distinct states that alternate in cycles and reflects differing levels of brain nerve cell activity. These are called REM sleep and non-REM sleep. During a normal night's sleep, everyone progresses through these stages five or six times:

Non-Rem Sleep

Non-Rapid Eye Movement Sleep (Non-REM) sleep is also termed quiet sleep. Non-REM sleep is is further subdivided into three stages of progression:
   o Stage 1 (light sleep).
   o Stage 2 (so-called true sleep).
   o Stage 3 to 4 (deep 'slow-wave' or delta sleep).

With each descending stage, awakening becomes more difficult. It is not known what governs Non-REM sleep in the brain, but it is believed that a balance between certain hormones, particularly growth and stress hormones may be important for deep sleep.

REM Sleep

Rapid Eye-Movement Sleep (REM) sleep is termed active sleep and most vivid dreams occur during this stage. REM-sleep brain activity is comparable to that in waking, but the muscles are virtually paralysed, possibly preventing us from acting out the dreams. In fact, except for vital organs like lungs and heart, the only muscles *not* paralysed during REM are the eye muscles. REM sleep may be critical for learning and for day-to-day mood regulation. When people are sleep-deprived, their waking brains have to work harder than when they are well rested.

The cycle between quiet (Non-REM) and active (REM) sleep generally follows the same pattern. After about 90 minutes of Non-REM sleep, eyes move rapidly behind closed lids, giving rise to REM sleep. As sleep progresses the Non-REM/REM cycle repeats. With each cycle, Non-REM sleep becomes progressively lighter, and REM sleep becomes progressively longer, lasting from a few minutes early in sleep to perhaps an hour at the end of the sleep episode.

What controls sleep?

In order to help change sleep patterns it is therefore necessary to understand the process which controls sleep. There are three processes which control sleep – the sleep system, the awake system and the biological clock. Sleep is not just a process of letting go. Rather, it is these three processes acting together – sleep takes over more and more of the brain, and the awake process decreases in grip.

The biological clock appears to exert some control over the awake process. It can cause certain disorders when it runs at the wrong speed, making people go to bed later and later (adolescence and young people are more prone), or earlier and earlier (older people have more problems with this). The clock can also run just slightly at the wrong pace, or the cues that synchronise it may not exert a strong effect. Cues include light, feeding, physical activity, work or social activity. One reason that elderly people may go to bed progressively earlier and earlier is that they do not go outside enough, or get enough natural light from windows, to help keep their biological clock set at the right time.

Your own unique pattern

Sleep is therefore pattern-based. How much sleep we need varies from person to person (there is no right or wrong answer to how much sleep you need). No matter how unusual your pattern, your body will work to maintain that pattern.

Some people prefer to work later, go to bed late and wake up late. These people are referred to as 'Owls'. Others are just the opposite, preferring to get up early and go to bed early. These people are called 'Larks'.

The important point is that if Owls go to bed late, too soon relative to their clocks, they will spend a long time going to sleep. Also if they have to get up early, between 6-8am in the morning, they will end up feeling as if they have not slept well enough. If this goes on for a while they could well end up thinking they are insomniacs, when all that is happening is that they are fighting against their own natural rhythms.

Larks could try and force themselves to stay up later in the evenings, but are still likely to wake up early. Again they too could misunderstand the situation and believe that they have a sleep problem.

Over to you - Understanding your Sleep patterns

Think about and record in your notebook or journal:

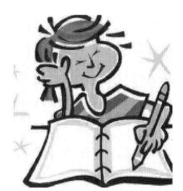

1. What processes control sleep?

2. Are you an Owl or a Lark?

3. Name some of the factors that have an effect on your sleep:

4. How long you think you might have slept for?

5. How long it took you to fall asleep?

6. How many times you woke up?

Chapter 4:

ALL ABOUT INSOMNIA

Insomnia is the sensation of daytime fatigue and impaired performance caused by insufficient sleep. In general, people with insomnia experience one or more of the following:

- an inability to sleep despite being tired
- a light, fitful sleep that leaves them fatigued upon awakening
- waking up too early

Under debate is the question of whether insomnia is always a symptom of some other physical or psychological condition or whether in some cases it is a primary disorder of its own. Common symptoms of insomnia include:

- feeling tired during the day
- irritability
- lack of concentration

- Waking up feeling tired and not refreshed
- sleeping better away from home
- taking longer than 30 or 40 minutes to fall asleep
- waking repeatedly during the night
- waking far too early and being unable to fall back asleep
- being able to sleep only with the aid of sleeping pills or alcohol

Insomniacs often complain of being unable to close their eyes or rest their minds for any period of time. This author certainly knows what it's like to have your mind racing at bedtime. In our stress-filled world, we are often plagued with unfinished to-do lists which run around in our heads. When it's quiet and time for sleep, many of us have problems pushing those to-do lists aside in favour of our dreams.

Often artistic types claim that they get their best ideas at night while lying in bed trying to sleep. One scholar even said that if a man had as many ideas during the day as he does when he has insomnia, he'd make a fortune. That may be true, but eventually, the lack of sleep will take its toll.

For many people, the worst part of insomnia is wanting to sleep, but being unable to. The mind races and is unable to rest and that makes you overly tired and barely able to function the next day. Chronic insomnia occurs when the following characteristics are present: When a person has difficulty falling asleep, maintaining sleep, or has non-restorative sleep for at least three nights a week for one month or longer. In addition, the patient is distressed and believes that normal daily functioning is impaired because of sleep loss. Secondary chronic insomnia is caused by medical conditions such as chronic pain or psychiatric conditions, drugs, or emotional or psychiatric disorders.

What causes insomnia?

While there is no one cut and dried reason why some people can't sleep, most experts agree that insomnia is brought on by stress, anxiety, pain, medications, and caffeine – among other things.

A reaction to change or stress is one of the most common causes of short-term insomnia. This condition is sometimes referred to as adjustment sleep disorder. The precipitating factor could be a major or traumatic event such as the following:
- An acute illness
- Injury or surgery
- The loss of a loved one
- Job loss
- Pain

Temporary insomnia could also develop after a relatively minor event, including the following:
- Extremes in weather
- An exam at school
- Travelling
- Trouble at work

In such cases, normal sleep almost always returns when the

condition resolves. Either the person affected recovers from the event, or they become used to the new situation. Treatment is needed only if sleepiness interferes with your everyday functioning or if the problem continues for more than a few weeks.

Female hormones
Fluctuations in female hormones play a major role in insomnia in women over their lifetimes. Such insomnia is most often temporary. The hormone progesterone promotes sleep. When they rise during ovulation, women may become sleepier than usual. During pregnancy, the effects of changes in progesterone levels in the first and last trimester can disrupt normal sleep patterns.

Levels of this hormone plunge during menstruation, causing insomnia. Insomnia can be a major problem in the first phases of menopause, when hormones are fluctuating intensely. Insomnia during this period may be due to different factors that occur. In some women, hot flushes, sweating, and a sense of anxiety can awaken them suddenly and frequently at night. In these cases, hormone replacement therapy may be beneficial. Insomnia may also be perpetuated by psychological distress provoked by this life passage. In most cases, insomnia is temporary. Cases of chronic insomnia in women over 50 are more likely to be due to other causes

Light
In one study, 20 percent of adults reported that light, noise, and uncomfortable temperatures caused their sleeplessness. Depending on the time of day too much or too little light can

disrupt sleep. It is well known that a person's biological circadian clock is triggered by sunlight and very bright artificial light may also cause wakefulness. One study indicated that even dim artificial light may disrupt sleep. Insufficient exposure to light during the day, as occurs in some disabled elderly patients who rarely venture outside, may also be linked with sleep disturbances. One study suggests that when a person is exposed to bright daylight, melatonin levels increase in response to darkness at night, which aids sleep.

Stimulants
Caffeine most commonly disrupts sleep. Nicotine can cause wakefulness. Quitting smoking can also cause transient insomnia. In fact, it has been suggested that if sleeping could be improved during withdrawal from smoking, then perhaps it would be easier to quit smoking.

Snoring
Your partner's sleep habits can also cause insomnia. In one 1999 survey, 17 percent of women and 5 percent of men reported that their partner's sleep habits impaired their own sleep. Snoring can certainly be a factor in a partner's insomnia. In fact, in the same survey 44 percent of men and 36 percent of women reported snoring a few nights a week and of those who snored, 19 percent could be heard through a closed door.

Medication
Insomnia is a side effect of many common medications, including over-the-counter preparations that contain caffeine. People who suspect their medications are causing them to lose sleep should check with your GP or pharmacist.

Underlying causes

Chronic insomnia can also have deep seated roots. In many cases, it is unclear if chronic insomnia is a symptom of some physical or psychological condition or if it is a primary disorder of its own. In most instances, a collaboration of psychological and physical conditions causes the failure to sleep. Psycho-physiologic insomnia is the revolving door of sleeplessness:

- An episode of transient insomnia disrupts the person's circadian rhythm
- The patient begins to associate the bed not with rest and relaxation but with a struggle to sleep. A pattern of sleep failure emerges
- Overtime, this event repeats, and bedtime becomes a source of anxiety. Once in bed, the patient broods over the inability to sleep and the loss of mental control. All attempts to sleep fail
- After such a cycle is established, insomnia becomes a self-fulfilling prophecy that can persist indefinitely

Sometimes anxiety and the inability to sleep dates back to childhood when parents used various threats to force their children into sleep for which they may not have been ready.

As you are aware, pain and discomfort from an injury, illness, or disability can also impair sleep. Among the many medical problems that can cause insomnia are: allergies, arthritis, cancer, heart disease, gastro reflux disease, hypertension, and asthma. When people are in pain or sick, generally they have medication to help them through the uncomfortable symptoms. Unfortunately, many of these medicines can also cause insomnia to onset or worsen. Medicines which can cause problems include some anti-depressants and beta-blockers. A large percentage of chronic insomnia cases prove to have a psychological or even psychiatric basis. Anxiety, depression, and bipolar disorder are the most common culprits. On top of that, insomnia may cause emotional problems, and it is often unclear which condition has triggered the other, or if the two conditions, in fact, have a common source.

Anxiety
Anxiety accounts for almost 50 percent of the cases of chronic insomnia. Feeling uptight and anxious can keep you from relaxing enough to go to sleep. A national survey by the US Department of Health and Human Services found that 47 percent of those reporting severe insomnia also reported feeling a high level of emotional distress. It could be that you become so tense and restless during a hard day at work that you don't even expect to sleep well at night.

Substance abuse
An estimated 10 percent to 15 percent of chronic insomnia cases result from substance abuse, especially alcohol, and sedatives. One or two alcoholic drinks at dinner, for most people, pose little danger of alcoholism and may help reduce stress and initiate sleep. Excess alcohol or alcohol used to promote sleep, however, tends to fragment sleep and cause wakefulness a few hours later.

Stress hormones
Persistently high levels of stress hormones, particularly cortisol,

may be key factors in many cases of chronic insomnia, particularly insomnia related to aging and psychiatric disorders. High levels of cortisol reduce REM sleep. Abnormal levels of other biologic factors may also a play a role in specific situations.

Ageing
An imbalance in specific hormones important in sleep has been associated with ageing and may be partly responsible for the higher incidence of insomnia in older people. Older people experience higher levels of major stress hormones (cortisol and adrenocorticotropin) during the night. Why is this?

Normal ageing is associated with a blunting of regular, cyclical surges of growth hormone. This hormone, which is normally secreted in the late night, is associated not only with growth but with deep, slow-wave sleep. Older people generally have less slow-wave sleep.

Melatonin levels, the hormone secreted by the pineal gland are lower, in older people. Some research suggests that elderly people may have lower levels in general simply because many stay mostly indoors and out of normal sunlight. In spite of such observations a number of studies report no higher risk for insomnia in older adults who have no accompanying mental or physical problems.

There may also be a genetic link to insomnia. Sleep problems seem to run in families; approximately 35 percent of people with insomnia have a family history of the problem, with the mother being the most commonly affected family member. Still, because so many factors are involved in insomnia, a genetic component is difficult to define.

So we've seen that there can be many reasons why some people simply cannot sleep. Does this disorder affect certain people more than others?

Diagnosing insomnia

It might be helpful for you if we look at the basic sleep patterns and how doctors are able to identify specific problems based on what they already know about sleep. Diagnosing sleep disturbance and its cause is the most important step in restoring healthy sleep. There is little agreement, even among experts, however, on the best methods for effectively assessing a patient's insomnia.

A major difficulty in diagnosing this problem is its subjective nature. People who believe they have insomnia may have actually had frequent brief awakenings during sleep that they perceive as being continuously awake. A number of questionnaires are available for determining whether a person has insomnia or other sleep disorders. For example, you may get asked the following questions:

- How would your sleep problem be described?
- How long has your sleep problem been experienced?
- How long does it take you to fall asleep?
- How many times a week does it occur?
- How restful is your sleep?

○ Does the difficulty lie in getting to sleep or in waking up early?

○ What is your sleep environment like (Noisy? Not dark enough?)?

○ How does insomnia affect your daytime functioning?

○ What medications are you taking (including the use of self-medications for insomnia, such as herbs, alcohol, and over-the-counter or prescription drugs)?

○ Are you taking or withdrawing from stimulants, such as coffee or tobacco?

○ How much alcohol do you consume per day?

○ What stresses or emotional factors may be present in your life?

○ Have you experienced any significant life changes?

○ Do you snore or gasp during sleep (this could be an indication of sleep apnoea)?

○ Do you have leg problems (cramps, twitching, crawling feelings)?

○ If you have a bed partner, is his or her behaviour distressing or disturbing?

○ Are you a shift worker? Now or in the past?

Over to you – Your sleep diary

For the purpose of getting the most from this book, I

would suggest that you keep

a sleep diary to keep track of

your sleeping habits in your

notebook or journal. Every

day for at least 6 weeks, you

should record all sleep-

related information, including responses to questions

listed above described on a daily basis. A bed partner (if

you have one) can help by adding his or her observations

of your sleep behaviour.

Here's what you should include in your sleep diary to look

at your sleep pattern:

sleeping with pain

1. What time did you wake up this morning?

2. What time did you get up from bed this morning?

3. What time did you go to bed last night?

4. What time did you put the light out?

5. How long did it take you to get to fall asleep?

6. How many times did you wake in the night?

7. How long were you awake during the night?

8. How long did you sleep altogether?

9. How much alcohol did you have last night?

10. How many sleeping pills did you take last night?

11. Thinking about the quality of your sleep, record your answers to these questions: On a scale of 0-4, 0=not at all, 4=very good

12. How well rested do you feel this morning?

13. Was your sleep of good quality?

PART TWO - MOVING FORWARD - strategies for restful sleep

We have spent time in previous chapters to increase our knowledge of pain, sleep and insomnia, so now it's time to start to discuss practical ways that might improve your sleep.

sleeping with pain

Chapter 5

SLEEP HYGIENE: healthy lifestyle and good routines

Sleep hygiene conveys the idea of the 'sleep basics' and consists of two parts. The first part refers to things about your lifestyle and the second part, your preparation for bed that if changed, might improve your sleep pattern. Although you may not be aware, your lifestyle will have a huge effect on your sleep.

Sleep hygiene *refers to sleep habits and conditions which promote sleep as opposed to habits which do not. Obvious bad habits are drinking alcohol or caffeine in the evening, these make it hard for you to unwind and get to sleep.*

Sleep hygiene *should be your first line of attack against insomnia, and it is often used in conjunction with stimulus control and cognitive behaviour restructuring (see below). So a* *good start is to review your habits and make some changes in your routine to see if behavioural and environmental changes improve your sleep.*

Here are some tips for effective sleep hygiene habits in terms of lifestyle:

- *Establish a regular time for going to bed and getting up in the morning and stick to it even on weekends and during holidays.*
- *Use the bed for sleep and sexual relations only, not for reading, watching television, or working; excessive time in bed seems to fragment sleep.*
- *Avoid naps, especially in the evening.*
- *Exercise before dinner. A low point in energy occurs a few hours after exercise; sleep will then come more easily. If you exercise too close to bedtime, this may increase alertness.*
- *Take a hot bath about an hour and a half to two hours before bedtime. This alters the body's core temperature rhythm and helps people fall asleep more easily and more continuously. (Taking a bath shortly before bed increases alertness.)*
- *Do something relaxing in the half-hour before bedtime. Reading, meditation, colouring, listening to relaxing music are all appropriate activities.*
- *Keep the bedroom relatively cool and well ventilated.*
- *Do not look at the clock. Obsessing over time will just make it more difficult to sleep.*
- *Eat light meals and schedule dinner four to five hours before bedtime. A light snack before bedtime can help*

sleep, but a large meal may have the opposite effect.

- *Avoid fluids just before bedtime so that sleep is not disturbed by the need to urinate.*
- *Avoid caffeine or other stimulants, such as nicotine in the hours before sleep. A general recommendation is not to consume anything that might hinder your sleep 4-6 hours before your anticipated bedtime.*
- *Don't drink alcohol before going to bed.*
- *If you are still awake after 15 or 20 minutes go into another room, read or do a quiet activity using dim lighting until feeling very sleepy. (Don't watch television or use bright lights.)*
- *Give yourself a quiet time right before bed. Just before you retire, take a few moments to spend quietly relaxing and meditating.*
- *If distracted by a sleeping bed partner, moving to the couch or a spare bed for a couple of nights might be helpful.*
- *Switch off your smartphone or tablet as they emit blue light which mimics daylight and can fool our internal body clocks.*

If you can't sleep -- don't stay in bed. Get out of bed, move to another room, and return to your bed when you are tired.

CASE STUDY Mrs A cuts out cigarettes and coffee

Mrs A, was a 55-year-old married lady who suffered with insomnia brought on by chronic pain. She reported a 10-year history of chronic pain following an accident at work. She has a 7-year history of problems with her sleeping, mainly that once she got comfortable she would get off to sleep but a couple of hours later, she would wake and not be able to get back to sleep.

We discussed basic sleep hygiene and it emerged that Mrs A drank 8 -10 coffees per day and smoked 60 cigarettes most days. As our conversation evolved, it became apparent that when Mrs A couldn't sleep, she would get up and have a coffee and a cigarette.

Following further conversation, Mrs A decided that for the next week she would reduce her caffeine intake to 4-5 cups of coffee a day and that she would not smoke after 8pm (her usual bedtime was about 11.30pm) if she got up in the night she would have a hot chocolate drink and not smoke during this time.

We met again approximately 10 days later, Mrs A assures me that she stuck to her plan and reported waking and having to get up only twice during the night rather than her usual five or six times per night. She was really pleased with this and agreed next, to reduce her nicotine intake.

This was more challenging for her, after two weeks she had managed to cut down to 20 per day and reported sleeping so much better and for longer, on average waking only twice briefly and she could easily get back to sleep. She reported that she actually felt as if she had slept.

CASE STUDY Mr B changes his mattress

Mr B is a gentleman in his late 70's and reported that his back and leg pain made it extremely difficult to get comfortable in order to get to sleep.

We discussed basic sleep hygiene and he identified that he thought that his mattress was about 20 years old and wasn't sure about the age of his pillows!

He was in the financial position that he could afford to change his mattress and pillows. We discussed the importance of feeling comfortable in bed, so when he went to choose one I suggested that he spent at least 10 minutes lying and sitting on each mattress. He was a little concerned about this, so following further discussion; he decided to go to the shop on a weekday morning when there were less customers, so he didn't feel quite so awkward.

Approximately a month later, we met again and he told me that he had gone into the shop when it was quiet and explained to the salesman that he had a bad back. He reports that the salesman was excellent and suggested mattresses that might be suitable and he brought various pillows over for this gentleman to try whilst he was trying out the mattresses.

He also told me that once he thought he had found a suitable pillow and mattress the salesman left him alone to try it out. Mr B purchased that particular combination and after a few days of getting used to it found it was taking much less time to get to sleep.

He reported that sometimes his leg would be extra painful if he had done a little too much, so I suggested that he place a pillow between his knees. This seems to be a winning combination for Mr B as he reports that he now is able to get to sleep within 10 minutes of his head touching the pillow, which is great.

Over to you – do you need to make adjustments to your sleep hygiene?

Make a note of your answers in your notebook or journal.

1) Make a list of all the things you think have caffeine in them – you will be surprised at how many there are!

2) Do you think your lifestyle could be improved to help you sleep?

3) Write down any decisions you have made about each of those lifestyle areas.

Remember to keep recording your sleep as suggested in part 1, chapter 5.

sleeping with pain

Chapter 6

GOAL SETTING: solve the insomnia problem!

In order to understand sleep it is important to recognise that sleep is an active process, the body's processes during sleep are vital to life. For example, it is during sleep that our body tissue is repaired.

Sleep is made up of different subtypes and stages as well as being orderly. As these types and stages are organised in a series of cycles, they repeat across the night. You may have noticed that variations in your sleep patterns have altered your cycle, changing many aspects of your life including how you feel and behave.

Now is the time to take control and change any self-defeating perspectives that leave you feeling powerless, and instead start to view insomnia as a problem that can be solved! By changing how you perceive insomnia and altering specific behaviours, you can reduce sleep disruptions. It is important to consider your thoughts and feelings surrounding sleep and sleeplessness clearly and accurately. By spending time focusing on your thoughts you can record, evaluate and reassess your perception of sleep, as well as develop a NEW way of thinking.

The challenge of change is not so daunting if we think about it *in terms of changing just one small aspect of behaviour*. So how do we do this? By GOAL SETTING.

Setting goals is a crucially important skill, planning properly greatly enhances the chances of success!

When thinking about setting goals remember these criteria:

1. **A goal should be measurable** – can you tell when your goal has been reached?
2. **A goal should be realistic** – is it possible to achieve, even when you are in pain?
3. **A goal should be behavioural** – does it involve specific actions or steps to take?
4. **A goal should be "I" centred** – are you the one taking part in the actions or behaviours being measured?
5. **A goal should be desirable** – do you want the outcome enough to put in the effort required

In order to make meaningful goals we need to clearly state:
   ○ What we want
   ○ How we are going to get it
   ○ How long it is going to take

These factors are definite, objective and visible; a clear goal should have all 3 of these things.

Here is an example:
- **Goal** - I will sleep for more than four hours each night
- **How** – By looking at my sleep environment and seeing what I could change
- **Timeline** – I'm going to achieve this at least once by the end of the programme.

It cannot be said too often, that working on personal goals is never easy. There are a thousand distractions and excuses we can find for putting off the day which we start to take control. Setting proper goals is good self-discipline. After all, if change didn't require self-discipline, we would have worked things out by now.

CASE STUDY Mrs M stays awake

Mrs M is a 45-year-old employed lady with chronic low back pain. She had reduced her hours at work due to her pain. Her job involved admin so she was sitting down most of the time she was at work.

After work she would come home and sit watching TV and often fell asleep until her husband got home. At bedtime, she would find it difficult to get to sleep and often stay up late, doze on the sofa before eventually getting to bed at 3 am. This pattern she felt made her pain worse and she was experiencing daytime fatigue.

We spent time discussing basic sleep hygiene and the importance of exercise. She readily accepted the idea of exercise once I had explained I didn't expect her to join a gym, walking would be fine! We discussed the concept of the association between sleep and bed, so she needed to avoid taking naps in the chair (see chapter 9 for more on this).

This was her goal:

GOAL: I will not fall asleep in the afternoon after work

HOW: I will sit down for an hour when I get home from work. I will set an alarm if needs be. Then I will have a short walk, then sit down for an hour, before starting to prepare dinner.

TIMESCALE: I am going to do this every weekday for 2 weeks and then reassess if it has any impact on my sleeping patterns.

Results: Mrs M found this difficult some days. She did find that setting an alarm for 30 minutes, stopped her from napping or woke her on the days she found herself nodding off. She found that she started looking forward to her walk and regularly met one of her neighbours who was usually out walking their dog so would strike up a conversation and fuss the dog!

At our next consultation, Mrs M was keen to be walking a little further so we discussed the concept of pacing, so she could adapt and start to walk further without causing a flare up of her pain.

With regards to her sleep, since adding the walking and avoiding napping in the afternoon has found that her sleep has started to improve.

Mrs M is happier that she now goes to bed at the same time as her husband, so doesn't have to worry about disturbing him when coming to bed. Mrs M tells me that now she has a reason to go out in the afternoon she feels she is less fatigued. She reports that she found goal setting a useful tool and is applying it to other areas of her life to help her manage her pain more effectively.

Over to you: a template for goal setting

To help regain control of
your life, you may need to
change your behaviour. This
seems like a daunting task
but if we think of it as
changing one aspect of

behaviour it is easier to deal with. We can do this by
GOAL SETTING.

A) What five criteria should you remember when setting
goals?

1)

2)

3)

4)

5)

Over to you: a template for goal setting

B) *In order to set meaningful goals what three things do we need to state clearly?*

1)

2)

3)

C) Why is it important to go through the above steps for goal setting?

D) Write down three goals for yourself in your journal or notebook.

E) Now split the goal which has greatest priority for you into how and timeline.

Remember to keep a record of your sleep in your notebook or journal

sleeping with pain

Chapter 7

CHANGING OUR OWN THOUGHTS ABOUT SLEEP

So now we have learnt to set a goal in relation to improving our sleep, we need to consider insomnia as a problem that can be solved!

It is about acknowledging that insomnia is frustrating and annoying, but your negative thoughts towards it won't change it. In this next chapter, we are going to look at how we can challenge those negative thoughts, emotions and beliefs about your sleep and put you back in control. As I have said earlier, sleep is a learned behaviour, so we know that you can learn to sleep better!

Below describes the role of thoughts and feelings and the part they play in the whole process of managing your pain and sleep.

It's important that we learn to recognise the effects of situations on our feelings. We all know that certain situations will produce certain emotions or feelings within us. For example, being let down by someone can make you feel sad or angry or frustrated. Achieving a personal goal may make you feel happy, successful and positive about tackling your next goal.

Long-term health conditions, such as chronic pain and lack of sleep, produce a whole range of feelings, both positive and negative. As you readjust to what you have been through, you can experience frustration and disappointment which must be expected at times. Our feelings and emotions produce certain types of thinking. Negative thinking emotions such as frustration, anger, helplessness tend to produce negative thoughts such as:

"I can't cope without sleep"

"There is nothing that will help me out"

"My sleep is never going to get any better"

"I ought to be able to cope with this"

"I must get myself on top of all these problems"

These negative thoughts are very destructive. They can put a lot of pressure on you. For example, if you tell yourself "I should be able to cope" you could push yourself and this could make your pain and sleep worse.

Negative thoughts such as those below can also stop you using your strategies such as relaxation and pacing.

"I haven't slept all night, so I can't do anything today"

"I haven't slept very much and I'm in too much pain to go for a walk, so I won't be able to go out today"

Negative thinking will stop positive action . . . what can YOU do with negative thinking?

- ○ Firstly, **RECOGNISE** your negative thought "I haven't had any sleep, everyone else sleeps well";

- ○ **NOTICE HOW THIS MAKES YOU FEEL**- anxious, annoyed, jealous

- ○ **THINK POSITIVELY BUT REALISTICALLY**- "Although it feels like I haven't had any sleep, in reality I probably have had some sleep if I look in my sleep diary. I know other people who have pain and don't sleep well, so everyone isn't sleeping!"

- ○ **NOTICE HOW THIS MAKES YOU FEEL**- less annoyed, reassured, more optimistic

It's important to catch these negative thoughts as they occur and challenge them with positive but realistic statements.

Positive thinking puts YOU in control of your situation. Once you start thinking positively, then it becomes easier to try all the practical things that will help with your pain and sleep.

Negative thinking stops you from taking control and often ends up making you feel worse.

It would be beneficial for you to take a little time and write down your negative thought in your notebook or journal and begin to challenge them in a realistic and positive way.

Negative thoughts create a vicious cycle; they stop you from taking positive action, which feeds into negative feeling or emotions and proves the negative thoughts to be true.

CASE STUDY Mr C uses his diary

Mr C was a 43-year-old gentleman who presented with chronic low back pain, anxiety and insomnia. We discussed his anxiety which was made worse by not sleeping. "I haven't slept in over 2 weeks" and he reported feeling anxious and frustrated because of his lack of sleep.

I asked Mr C to look back in his notebook and look at his sleep diary for evidence of whether or not he has slept. Looking at the entries on his sleep diaries, it appeared that he had some sleep albeit he didn't think it was enough. So by looking at the diaries, asking what's the evidence that Mr C hadn't slept for two weeks? We found that he had slept for a few hours most nights. I asked him, that knowing that he was starting to improve the amount of sleep; was he now feeling less anxious and frustrated about sleeping and not getting to sleep. He reported that he had found it a helpful exercise to start to challenge his negative thoughts.

Our next appointment was a few weeks later, when Mr C reported that he had written a list of positive self-statements on a card and kept them on his bedside table. So rather than get frustrated, he would challenge his negative thoughts and found that he was getting to sleep within 15 minutes and maintaining that until 5-6 am, which he felt was acceptable.

Over to you – what are your negative thoughts?

Consider the following questions when considering challenging your negative thoughts.

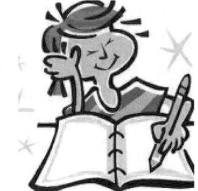

1. Am I confusing a thought with a fact? (what is the evidence?)

2. Am I jumping to conclusions?

3. Am I asking questions that have no answers?

4. Am I thinking in all or nothing terms? (always/ never/nothing/everything)

5. Am I concentrating on my weaknesses rather than my strengths?

6. Am I expecting myself to be perfect?

7. Am I overestimating the chances of disaster?

Over to you – what are your negative thoughts?

8. Am I exaggerating the importance of events?

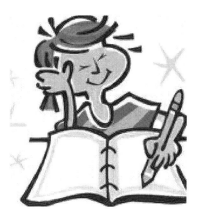

9. Am I fretting about the way things ought to be, or how I wish they were?

10. Am I predicting the future instead of experimenting with it?

At first, you may find it hard to begin using positive statements. However as with any new skill, practice makes perfect and with time, you will begin to feel the benefits of breaking the negative cycle and start to feel and sleep better.

Over to you – what are your negative thoughts?

Here are some positive self- statements to help get you started:

"Almost certainly I will get some sleep"

"I know other people with pain who don't sleep well too"

"There are lots of factors, not just lack of sleep that makes my pain worse"

"When looking in my notebook/ journal, I usually average 5 hours, never less than 3"

Remember to keep recording your sleep as suggested in part 1, chapter 5

Chapter 8

PROGRAMMING YOUR SLEEP PATTERNS

So you have set your goal, changed the way you see your insomnia and feel that it is something you can tackle and it will improve, read on! In this chapter we aim to re-programme your sleep pattern so that you develop a strong and lasting sleep pattern that meets your requirements.

Be prepared for some tough stuff. The work in this chapter is the hardest bit. You have to be ready to make the changes and be committed to following them through the best you can, even when it feels very hard. It will get easier with time and the strategies in the next chapters will help. You may relapse, but don't worry, don't be put off, just get back on track the next day.

Most importantly we need to consider the connection between your sleep and your bed. The majority of good sleepers associated their bed with sleep. Those who don't sleep well such as yourself, will associate their bed with frustration, lying awake tossing and turning, noticing high levels of pain and being unable to get comfortable. These thoughts often produce feelings of anxiety which stimulate the pain system thus increasing pain and not being able to sleep and so the cycle continues.

Sleep is a learned behaviour. This means we can make a response to a cue, and the cue will be your bed. It will become quicker and be easier for you to fall asleep and go back to sleep. When you wake your body associates your bed (cue) with sleep (learned behaviour). It is important to strengthen that cue (your bed) and sleep, so you will need to follow some rules.

In order to develop that strong link between your bed and sleep, it's really important not to use your bed for anything except sleep. You need to avoid doing things that you would do when you are awake such as watching TV, reading, eating, studying, using the phone and chatting to friends on social media. The rationale is that if you use your bed for activities other than sleep, you are training yourself to stay awake in bed. If you avoid these activities, over time your bed will become a place where it is easy to go to sleep and stay asleep. Sex is the only exception to this rule; it might even help your sleep afterwards!

As soon as you get into bed, immediately turn out the light and put your head on the pillow as it is your intention to sleep. The reason for this is that you need to learn to fall asleep very quickly after you get in bed. While in bed, don't mull over your problems or plan future events, even what's happening tomorrow. Over-thinking sets your mind racing which is a bad habit to get into. (Some advice on dealing with stopping your thoughts running around is in a later chapter).

If you are not asleep within 15 minutes of going to bed, get up and go into another room and do something. This is important because it promotes your sleep/bed connection, in that in bed, you sleep, it also keeps being awake associated with things that you do when you are awake and not in bed.

I appreciate that getting up during the night is difficult, especially when it's cold! If possible, perhaps you could keep your heating on low; perhaps have a flask of a warm drink made up. You could spend time reading, or maybe listening to gentle music, or watching something gentle on TV, no adrenaline filled action movies! Spending time on such activities avoids you lying in bed becoming more and more frustrated.

After this first time, you don't have to count down the clock for 15 minutes before you get up again and if you cannot sleep, you can get up whenever you like. This will avoid the frustration of clock watching.

Please don't be fed up and disheartened if at first you are up and down quite a few times each night when you start doing this . . . this is normal.

It is important to go only to bed when you are 'sleepy-tired' that is when you get itchy eyes, lack of energy, start yawning, muscles feel tired and you start to nod off. Sleepiness rather than tiredness is a signal that it is time for our night of sleep.

Make sure you do not go to bed too early for you, or you will find yourself spending far more time in bed than what you need for sleep. Spending too much time in bed often results in a very broken night's sleep and weakens the bed/sleep association.

Remember daytime is for being awake, so avoid napping

throughout the day or early evening if possible. This is another way of reinforcing the association that bed is for sleep, and night time is for sleeping. Napping in the chair weakens the connection between bed and sleep. If you really, really have to have a nap, then make sure it's no longer than 15 minutes and is before 3.00pm.

RECAP OF THE RULES

1. Bed is only for sleeping

2. Get up if you can't sleep

3. Only go to bed when you are sleepy-tired

4. Avoid napping in the daytime

5. Do not worry, plan or problem solve in bed

The next thing to consider is how much sleep do we need? I'm sure this will be different to how much sleep you want!

As outlined in the first part of this book, our sleep requirements change throughout our lives, so we have to adapt accordingly.

Our sleep can be different each night, sometimes we sleep through for five hours, at other times our sleep is broken so it feels like we haven't had enough sleep. Your sleep was probably like this before you had chronic pain.

This book aims to help to reduce the difficulty in getting to sleep and improve your ability to stay asleep and the following chapters will help you with this. As I said at the beginning of this book, don't pick and choose the ones you like best, try them all for best results!

Over to you. Get a new pattern in place over time

Jot down your answers to these questions in your notebook or journal.

1.What decisions have I made about bedtime activities?

2.What decisions have I made about the 15 minute rule?

3.What activities have I planned if I get up because I can't sleep?

4.How am I going to avoid napping in the daytime / early evening?

5.How will I know when I'm sleepy rather than tired or fatigued?

In your notebook or journal turn back to your sleep diary entries as we can use these, to find out how much sleep you really need; you should have quite a few now.

1) Write down the total time you think you actually slept in the past 10 days.

2) Next add up the total time that you have slept across these nights.

3) Then divide the total by 10 to get the average length of a night's sleep.

Don't worry if you have come up with a figure less than the amount of sleep you are aiming for, this is just the beginning! Remember, this book aims to help to reduce the difficulty in getting to sleep and improve your ability to stay asleep. We can build up your total sleep time to the amount you need. Remember to keep recording your sleep. (Go back to Part 1, chapter 5 to remind yourself how to do this)

Over to you. When should I go to bed and when should I get up?

Now we have decided how much sleep we need, our next

challenge is to work out how

to get the same amount of

sleep every night. This is

important as we are aiming

for you to sleep through this

period without waking, thus

producing a stable sleep pattern.

It is important for you to set yourself a time that you will

get up in the morning. This time will be the same every

morning, even at weekends! Choose a time that suits you

and that you will be able to stick to.

Now you have a fixed time to get up in the morning and

your average sleep time.

When you feel sleepy-tired is the best time for you to go to bed as there is more chance you will sleep for longer. Next we need to consider your threshold time; this is the earliest time you can consider going to bed if you are sleepy-tired, not your actual bedtime as such.

To work out your threshold time, you need to subtract your average sleep time from your morning getting up time.

Here is an example. If your average sleep time is 6 hours, and you get up in the morning at 7.30am, 1.30am would be your threshold time. So you could go to bed any time after 1.30am as long as you are sleepy-tired.

Over to you. Recap

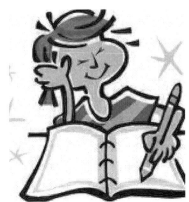

1. Stay up until your

threshold time

2. Lie down in bed only

when you feel sleepy

3. Do not use your bed for

anything other than sleep

4. If you don't get to sleep in 15 minutes, get up

5. If you still can't get to sleep, repeat step 4

6. If you wake during the night, repeat step 4.

7. Get up at your agreed time in the morning

8. Do not take naps throughout afternoon or evening

9. Follow this programme every day and night of the

week

A *word of encouragement*

As I said at the beginning of this chapter, this is tough! It is always difficult to make changes within our lives, even when we have chosen to change! It will take a great deal of extra effort to stick to your new schedule. Once you have started to sleep well, don't be tempted to stop applying all the knowledge you have learned and have been putting into practice as you have read this book. Only by maintaining your sleep patterns can they continue to be improved.

Relapses can happen as in all types of behaviour change! Please don't let this put you off; the best thing to do is to get back on track.

Once your sleeping begins to improve and you are getting to sleep quickly and staying asleep or easily getting back to sleep, you can start to increase gradually your time in bed, but remember all the rules still apply!

As your sleep starts to improve and you notice that you are sleeping 85 to 90 percent of the time between your threshold time and getting up in the morning most of the week, you can start slowly to add in more time in bed and hence sleep.

If you are achieving this, the following week you can add 15 minutes more, either by going to bed 15 minutes earlier or staying in bed an extra 15 minutes later. Try this out for a week and reassess to see if you are sleeping 85 to 90 percent of the time when in bed.

Please be strict with yourself and don't make changes bigger than 15 minutes each week. You can carry on with this until trying to be in bed for longer doesn't give you anymore sleep.

Continue to monitor your sleep in your notebook or journal as suggested in chapter 5 when discussing your sleep diary.

Over to you. Checklist

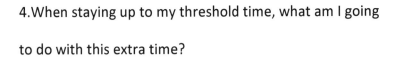

1.My fixed average sleep

time is?

2.I am going to get up in the

morning at?

3.My threshold time is?

4.When staying up to my threshold time, what am I going

to do with this extra time?

5.How do I recognise when I am sleepy?

6.As I can only use my bed for sleep, I will need to make

the following changes....

7.If I don't get to sleep within 15 minutes, when I get up,

what will I do?

8.Do I need to make any preparations before going to

bed?

9. If I still can't fall asleep when I go back to bed, what will I do?

10. If I wake up in the night, what exactly will I do?

11. How will I make sure that I will definitely get up at my allocated time?

12. How am I going to avoid taking naps throughout the day?

13. How will I manage to follow this programme for the next couple of weeks?

14. When I add 15 minutes extra on my sleep programme week, where will it be?

sleeping with pain

Chapter 9

TIPS FOR YOUR BEDTIME WIND DOWN

Although often we wish we could just fall asleep, it is unrealistic to think you can just fall into bed and then fall straight asleep.

By slowing down your activities 60-90 minutes before going to bed and having time to do other activities before bed, will help your body become more relaxed and on 'wind down' mode.

Some tips for bedtime wind down could include:
Approximately an hour before bed, sit down with a decaffeinated drink and a light snack and perhaps after a warm bath. You could read or watch TV, listen to music, do some mindful colouring or maybe or a combination of these. Learn to become a more relaxed person!! Most importantly **PLAN** your bedtime routine and stick to it every day.

For example
9.30 pm, have warm bath
10.00 pm, sit down with a decaffeinated drink and watch TV
10.30 pm, put the dog out, lock up, go upstairs, wash hands/face, clean teeth
11.00 pm, get into bed, do some gentle breathing exercise, fall asleep
As sleep is a learned behaviour, it is important to stick with the same routine every night.

Over to you: keep recording what works for you

Remember to keep recording your

sleep as suggested in part 1,

chapter 5

Chapter 10

STRESS MANAGEMENT AND RELAXATION

Learning to be physically and mentally relaxed before going to bed will help you fall asleep more quickly. Additionally, many relaxation techniques can be put to use when you wake up in the middle of the night and need to get back to sleep.

Relaxation has been described as: 'a feeling of refreshing tranquillity and an absence of tension or worry'. It is a state where tension among all the muscles in the body is absent, and it includes a state of mind in which stressors, negative self-talk, and other worries are eliminated from the mind.

There are two levels of relaxation.
●Deep Relaxation. Physical and mental tension are reduced to minimal levels
●Economy of effort. Tension is reduced to the level needed to maintain everyday activities.

To take an example, in your current circumstance, enjoying simple leisure activities may seem relaxing, but not relaxing enough. This is when implementing relaxation methods can help. Relaxation training and methods can increase a state of calmness and achieve that absence of tension or worry.

Quick Relaxation Technique
When faced with a difficult situation, and you feel your tension level rising, the following quick relaxation technique may help.
1. *Stop*
2. *Sigh*
3. *Drop your shoulders*
4. *Take two or three deeper, slower out breaths*
5. *Carry on more calmly and if possible, a little more slowly*

Learning to relax more deeply

Quieting your mind and body is not something that can be done immediately, so you should try to start winding down at least an hour before bed. Some people find that reading a book, taking a bath, playing solitaire or working a crossword puzzle are good ways to slow down from activity of the day. You may want to try one or more of the following activities:

Progressive Muscle Relaxation (PMR) – PMR is a set of exercises you can use to reduce anxiety and stress at bedtime. PMR is a two-step process where you first tense certain muscle groups and then relax them. As you go through the process, you should be focused on actively tensing and then relaxing, helping to relax your mind as well as your body. The procedure takes some time to learn, but after learning it, you can practice a shorter version of the exercises. When practising PMR to help with sleep, you should plan to fall asleep before finishing all of the exercises. (See the next chapter for a advice on PMR).

Diaphragmatic breathing Learning to breathe slowly and deeply from your belly or diaphragm is a good way to slow down. To practice belly breathing, put a hand on your stomach and take slow breaths, letting your stomach expand as you breathe in. As you breathe out, relax your chest and shoulders. Concentrate on your breathing as you do it to encourage your mind away from stressful or anxious thoughts.

Visual imagery relaxation Practising visual imagery means choosing peaceful, soothing thoughts to focus on which calm you and allow you to stop thinking of your 'to do' list. Everyone's peaceful situation is different, and you can choose to think about things that soothe *you* – a walk in the mountains, canoeing on a lake, swimming, petting your dog. As long as the image doesn't excite your mind, it should work.

Stress management If you learn to deal with stress more effectively through meditation or self-guided imagery, you should be able to fall asleep more easily. Try the following: Change or resolve the things causing you stress when possible.
  ○ Accept situations you can't change.
  ○ Keep your mind and body as relaxed as much as possible throughout the day.
  ○ Give yourself enough time to do the things you need to do - including eating.
  ○ Don't take on too much and avoid unrealistic demands.

- Live in the present, rather than worrying about the past or fearing the future.
- Talk to your partner if there are problems in your relationship.
- Have some relaxing, non-competitive activities - something you do just for pleasure, for fun.
- Give yourself some 'quiet time' each day.
- Practice a relaxation technique or breathing exercises.

Anger management Anger, anxiety and frustration can stand directly in the way of getting a good night's sleep. You may feel angry or anxious when you go to bed or you may become angry and frustrated when you can't go to sleep. Regardless of the source of the anger, recognise that it keeps your mind occupied and your body tense, two conditions which don't encourage sleep. A few things that might help you deal with your anger or anxiety:

- **Exercise daily** It will help you release excess anger and frustration. Think about the cause of your anger. If there isn't anything you can do to resolve it, move on. If you can resolve it, make steps to do so
- **Develop a method of releasing the anger** by the end of the day, before you try to relax or go to sleep. For example, you might choose to write it down in your journal or talk to a spouse or friend about it. After you have processed the anger and let it out, try to move on

Word and imagination games For some, playing mental games at bedtime may not be helpful at all. But others find that engaging their mind in something unimportant can be a good

way to unwind and shift attention away from actively trying to fall asleep. Try playing some mental games, for example:
- Spell long words and sentences backwards.
- Think of a poem or song and then count how many a's or b's there are in it. Work your way through the alphabet thinking of a four-letter word beginning with each letter
- Repeat long pieces of poetry or prose.
- Recall in great detail a favourite painting, a piece of music or place.

How self-help strategies work

These are usually effective and aren't addictive. Using these alternatives to over-the-counter or prescription medication are less expensive than pharmacological treatment, have fewer side effects, and can provide longer lasting relief particularly when behavioural treatments are used as well.

Use relaxation exercises to calm yourself and take your mind off of it. Take some diplomatic action to combat the noise that's disrupting your sleep. If your family is being noisy while you're trying to sleep, talk to them calmly about your need to sleep and ask them to please curtail the noise during bedtime hours.

Keep a radio or CD/MP3 player by your bed and use it to mask other noise. Try playing some relaxation music that can put you in a calmer mood and make you better able to cope with distractions. The most commonly identified benefits of relaxation are to:
- feel calmer, happier, and more energetic
- decrease heart rate, blood pressure, breathing rate

In the context of this book, relaxation can particularly benefit you in the following ways.

○ Relaxation can reduce pain. When muscle tension is reduced, certain aches and pains become less likely. e.g. headache, backache, cramp. Relaxation can increase an individuals' threshold for pain and lessen the perceived intensity of the pain.

○ Relaxation can reduce stress. Stress is an inevitable part of modern life and is increasingly being identified as detrimental to health. Relaxation is a key strategy in handling stress and attempts to counteract the bodily responses associated with stress.

The following table indicates the major body responses to stress and relaxation.

Stress Response		Relaxation Response
Up	Heart Rate	Down
Up	Blood Pressure	Down
Up	Breathing	Down
Up	Muscle tension	Down
Up	Sweating	Down
Up	State of mental arousal	Down
Up	Adrenaline Flow	Down

Regular practice of relaxation will help to minimise the harmful effects of stress. Relaxation can reduce fatigue by helping you gain deeper body awareness, and better judgement about the amount of effort you need to make for everyday tasks. Excessive and unnecessary tension (and therefore effort) is often employed in everyday activities. When economy of effort is employed, fatigue can be reduced. Relaxation can also promote sleep: when the body is resting peacefully and the mind is calm, sleep comes more easily. Relaxation can also improve self-confidence by increasing self-awareness, self-control and ability to cope; self-confidence can be improved. This in turn can increase performance in both work and leisure and improve the individual's ability to make and maintain social relationships.

Over to you: relaxation

Relaxation is a means of enabling physical or mental tension to be released. There are different levels to relaxation, deep relaxation and economy of effort.

1)What is deep relaxation?

2) What is economy of effort?

3)What are the five quick steps to relaxation?
1.
2.
3.
4.
5.

4) Relaxation can reduce the stress response. Name five major body responses to relaxation:
1.
2.
3.
4.
5.

5)What are the benefits of relaxation?

Chapter 11

PROGRESSIVE MUSCLE RELAXATION AND SELF-HYPNOSIS

One of the simplest and easily learned techniques for relaxation is Progressive Muscle Relaxation (PMR), a widely-used procedure today that was originally developed in 1939. The PMR procedure teaches you to relax your muscles through a two-step process.

First, you deliberately apply tension to certain muscle groups, and then you stop the tension and turn your attention to noticing how the muscles relax as the tension flows away. Through repetitive practice you quickly learn to recognize—and distinguish—the associated feelings of a tensed muscle and a completely relaxed muscle.

With this simple knowledge, you can then induce physical muscular relaxation at the first signs of the tension that accompanies anxiety.

And with physical relaxation comes mental calmness—in any

situation. Before practising PMR, you should consult with your doctor if you have a history of serious injuries, muscle spasms, or back problems, because the deliberate muscle tensing of the PMR procedure could exacerbate any of these pre-existing conditions. If you continue with this procedure against a doctor's advice, you do so at your own risk.

Two-step process
There are two steps in the self-administered Progressive Muscle Relaxation procedure: (a) deliberately tensing muscle groups, and (b) releasing the induced tension. This two-step process will be described after you are introduced to the muscle groups.

After learning the full PMR procedure as follows, you will spend about 10 minutes a day maintaining your proficiency by practising a shortened form of the procedure. As you practice the short procedure, you will be simultaneously learning cue-controlled relaxation.

Ultimately, you will acquire something that can become an indispensable part of your daily life and the initial drudgery of practice will be long-forgotten.

Regular practice
It is recommended that you practice full PMR twice a day for about a week before moving onto the shortened form (below). Of course, the time needed to master the full PMR procedure varies from person to person.

Before you start:

- ○ Always practice full PMR in a quiet place, along, with no distractions like television or phones. Don't use even background music.
- ○ Remove your shoes and wear loose clothing
- ○ Don't eat, smoke or drink right before practising PMR.
- ○ It's best to practice before meals rather than after to avoid problems with digestion.
- ○ Never practice this while under the influence of any intoxicants.
- ○ Sit in a comfortable chair or lying down in bed.
- ○ Plan on falling asleep before the cycle is complete if you do this in bed.
- ○ If you are doing PMR just to relax instead of falling asleep, after you are done, relax with your eyes closed for a few seconds and then get up slowly. If you stand up too quickly, you could experience a sudden drop in blood pressure which could cause you to feel faint.
- ○ Some people like to count backwards from 5 to 1 timed to slow, deep breathing and then say "Eyes open, supremely calm, fully alert."

You will be working with most of the major muscle groups in your body, but for convenience you will make a systematic progression from your feet upwards.

(Never listen to a PMR/CD/download whist driving a vehicle)

The recommended sequence:

Right foot
Right lower leg and foot
Entire right leg
Left foot
Left lower leg and foot
Entire left leg
Right hand
Right forearm and hand
Entire right arm
Left hand
Left forearm and hand
Entire left arm
Abdomen
Chest
Neck and shoulders
Face

If you're left handed, begin with your left side.

How to do it

Step One: Tension. The process of applying tension to a muscle is essentially the same regardless of which muscle group you are using. First, focus your mind on the muscle group; for example, your right hand. Then inhale and simply squeeze the muscles as hard as you can for about 8 seconds; (in the example, this would involve making a tight fist with your hand). Beginners usually make the mistake of allowing muscles other than the intended group to tense as well; in the example, this would be tensing muscles in your right arm and shoulder, not just in your right hand. With practice you will learn to make very fine discriminations among muscles; for the moment just do the best you can.

It can be difficult to achieve a fine degree of muscle separation when you start. Because neglect of the body is an almost universal cultural attitude, it is usually very difficult to begin learning how to take responsibility for your body's mechanics.

Take heart and realise that learning fine muscle distinction is in and of itself a major part of the overall PMR learning process. PMR isn't just about tension and relaxation – it's also about muscle discernment.

Relax and realize that no part of the body is an isolated unit. The muscles of the hand, for example, do have connections in the forearm, so when you tense your hand, there will still be some small tension occurring in the forearm.

When PMR asks that the hand be tensed without tensing the arm, it is really speaking to the beginner who, out of unfamiliarity with the body's muscles will unthinkingly tense everything in the whole arm. If you accept the fact that you are in the beginner phase and not inept at practicing the procedure, then you will begin to discover gently the fine muscles over time.

It's important really to feel the tension. Done properly, the tension procedure will cause the muscles to start to shake, and you will feel some pain.

Be careful not to hurt yourself, you should feel just mild pain. Contracting the muscles in your feet and your back, especially, can cause serious problems if not done carefully; that is gently but deliberately.

Step Two: Releasing the Tension. This is the best part because it is actually pleasurable. After the 8 seconds, just quickly and suddenly let go. Let all the tightness and pain flow out of the muscles as you simultaneously exhale.

Also imagine tightness and pain flowing out of your hand through your fingertips as you exhale. Feel the muscles relax and become loose and limp, tension flowing away like water out of a tap. Focus on this and notice the difference between tension and relaxation.

Notice the Difference. The point here is really to focus on the change that occurs as the tension is let go. Do this very deliberately, because you are trying to learn to make some very subtle distinctions between muscular tension and muscular relaxation.

Stay relaxed for about 15 seconds and then repeat this tension-relaxation cycle. You'll probably notice more sensations the second time.

Once you understand the muscle groups and the tension-relaxation procedure, then you are ready to begin the full PMR training. Simply follow the list of muscle groups in the sequence given and work through your entire body. Practice twice a day for a week. Spend extra time, if necessary, until you can achieve a deep sense of physical relaxation; then you can move onto the Shortened PMR schedule.

The shortened schedule

In the shortened form of PMR, you will work with summary groups of muscles rather than individual muscle groups, and begin to use cue-controlled relaxation.

The four summary muscle groups are:
Lower limbs
Abdomen and chest
Arms, shoulders, and neck
Face

Instead of working with just one specific part of your body at a time, simply focus on the complete group. In Group 1, for example, focus on both legs and feet all at once.

Cue-controlled relaxation:. Use the same tension-relaxation procedure as full PMR, but work with the summary groups of muscles. In addition, focus on your breathing during both tension and relaxation.

Inhale slowly as you apply and hold the tension. Then, when you let the tension go and exhale, say a cue word to yourself (below). This will help you to associate the cue word with a state of relaxation, so that eventually the cue word alone will produce a relaxed state.

Many people find that cue-controlled relaxation does not have to depend on only one word; it may actually be more helpful in some situations to use a particular phrase. Some suggestions for cue words/phrases include:

- Relax
- Let it go
- It's OK
- Stay calm
- All things are passing

Initially, you should practise the shortened form of PMR under the same conditions as you practised full PMR. After about a week of twice-daily practice you will then have enough proficiency to practise it under other conditions and with distractions. Or you might want to move onto the final process of Deep Muscle Relaxation.

Use anywhere
Once you have learned PMR and are familiar with the feeling of muscle relaxation, you can then induce relaxation without even bothering with the tension-relaxation process.

All you need to do is use your imagination to think of and then relax the various muscle groups using your cue word(s). Usually this is done by starting at the top of your head and then working down through your body, as if relaxation were being poured over your head and flowing down over all of your body. This process is called Deep Muscle Relaxation.

And, anywhere, anytime, you can simply perform a quick 'body scan' to recognise where in your body you might be holding muscle tension and then, using imagery and your cue word/phrase, let it go.

Self hypnosis

There are other approaches towards combating insomnia that can work well too. You may want to look into hypnosis for your sleeping problems or indeed to help you manage your pain. Self-hypnosis is especially helpful. This can be done either in person by consulting a psychologist or hypnotherapist who can devise a specific session for you. Or you may prefer to look online at many different sites that will allow you to download hypnotic sessions tailored to your specific problem. They are extremely relaxing and definitely worth the small investment! Equally you can use the scripts below:

Self-hypnosis script for sleep:
Lie down in your bed, ready for sleep and tell yourself that you are going to use self-hypnosis to help you go to sleep.

Close your eyes and begin to notice your breathing, slow, steady and even breaths. Breath in, count to three, exhale while counting to five. As you are breathing out imagine breathing out all your tension. You can also say the word 'relax' on each out breath if you like. Continue with this breathing pattern or 10 times or more until you feel totally relaxed.

Thinking about your breathing, but noticing the rise of your stomach as you breathe in and your stomach falling in as you breathe out (this is known as diaphragmatic breathing and it can take some practice).

Now, while you are carrying out you diaphragmatic breathing, think of the clouds in the sky and notice them drift past so your sky is clear, (and so is your mind of all conscious thoughts).

Next relax every muscle in your body from the top of your head to the tips of your toes, imagine them all relaxing, feeling soft, loose and relaxed. Notice that your eyelids are becoming heavier and heavier and your tension is disappearing.

Imagine this pattern of relaxation taking in your head, jaw, neck, shoulders, back, arms, abdomen and legs and feet. Imagine the feeling of relaxation trickling through your body getting rid of any tension. Visualise your muscles are being relaxed and concentrate on those areas of tension. Notice that your outside world is fading into the background.

When you are completely relaxed, you can say the following affirmations to yourself. It is important that you repeat these affirmations word for word. When you say these affirmations, really mean them and imagine yourself absorbing these affirmations with real belief and emotion.

I love to sleep at night
I sleep easily at night
I feel deeply relaxed
I feel calm and sleepy

At this point you can allow yourself to drift off into a deep and natural sleep.

Self–hypnosis script for pain:
Find a comfortable position and tell yourself that you are going to use self-hypnosis to help you control the level of your pain.

Close your eyes and begin to notice your breathing, slow, steady and even. Breath in, count to three, exhale while counting to five. As you are breathing out imagine breathing out all your tension. You can also say the word 'relax' on each out breath if you like. Continue with this breathing pattern for 10 times or more until you feel totally relaxed.

Thinking about your breathing, but noticing the rise of your stomach as you breathe in and your stomach falling in as you breathe out (this is known as diaphragmatic breathing and it can take some practice).

Next relax every muscle in your body from the top of your head to the tips of your toes, imagine them all relaxing, feeling soft, loose and relaxed. Notice that your eyelids are becoming heavier and heavier and your tension is disappearing. Imagine this pattern of relaxation taking in your head, jaw, neck, shoulders, back, arms, abdomen and legs and feet. Imagine the feeling of relaxation trickling through your body getting rid of any tension. Visualise your muscles are being relaxed and concentrate on those areas of tension. Notice that your outside world is fading into the background.

Now, visualise a dial on a control panel, it doesn't matter what the dial looks like. Notice the indicator on the dial, its hovering around a number that represents your current pain level. Notice that it's moving in time with your pain. Now, increase your pain just a little, but just enough so it registers on your dial, you notice the indicator moving.

You know you can increase your pain, do you know that you can make it decrease as well?

Focus on the indicator, focus on the number it is showing, and make your indicator easily move down, reducing your pain level so that the indicator is at a lower point than before and you are noticing that your pain has changed, has become less.

Now you have learned to control your pain and anytime you want to vary the level, you can use the indicator on your dial. You are in control and that is good to know.

When you are ready, open your eyes, have a gentle stretch, feeling confident that you can control your pain.

Over to you: choose and practice

In your notebook or journal,

consider these questions.

My chosen method is:

Will I record myself reading the instructions for my chosen

method?

When will I practice my relaxation or self-hypnosis?

What are the potential barriers that could prevent me

practicing my relaxation or self-hypnosis?

How can I overcome these barriers?

Chapter 12

STOPPING YOUR THOUGHTS RUNNING ROUND

People with insomnia complain a lot about an overactive mind in bed, which is why the busy and fast running mind is the enemy of sleep. By the end of this chapter you will have learned ways of overcoming the mental alertness, repetitive thoughts and anxieties that interfere with your sleep. Therefore let's consider the kinds of things that you think about when you are in bed and unable to sleep.

Paying attention to your body
This is when you focus inwards; you may notice how tired you are or different body sensations such as feeling too hot or a specific pain in your leg. These self-aware thoughts, when your mind is quite concentrated and focused make it even harder to get to sleep.

Thinking about sleep and not sleeping
When sleep doesn't come quickly and naturally, it is easy to become preoccupied with sleeplessness itself. Thinking about the fact that you cannot sleep, but you want to sleep, but you cannot stop thinking about wanting to sleep creates a vicious circle and often results in trying too hard to get to sleep.

Replaying thoughts and planning ahead
This is when you think back over the day, recent events or look ahead to up and coming occasions. Replaying the day's events is quite natural and sometimes enjoyable. Likewise is thinking of the day ahead and planning for the future. Re-hearing and planning thoughts might therefore keep you awake simply because they cause mental alertness in bed.

Problem-solving
This is when you have things on your mind as you think they 'need to get sorted out' so you stay awake while you try and come up with an answer. These thoughts require some concentrated attention because there maybe options to think through properly before a decision can be made. We then realise that we cannot think of a good solution which makes us even more mentally and emotionally alert.

Your mind is buzzing
This is when different thoughts which are trivial and unimportant causes frustration, because you know that what you are thinking about is unimportant and keeping you awake. Commonly, these thoughts may make you feel like you cannot control your thinking, even though you are not really worried about anything.

Feeling that control is slipping away is not good for relaxing into sleep.

Hearing noises in the night
Sometimes people cannot get to sleep because of the noises they hear or think they hear. E.g. The wind outside or people in the street, therefore your senses home in on what you have noticed.

Thoughts and feelings
Our mind is a combination of thoughts and feelings. Maybe you are worried about family or work so when you are having rehearsal or planning type thoughts you may get strong emotional feelings. Thoughts plus feelings therefore keep you even more awake.

Over to you: thoughts that keep you awake

It is useful for you to review your responses every few weeks, so you can focus on the areas you need to work on and see you progress! These questions are based on The Glasgow Content of Thought Scale.

1. Am I worrying about events that happened today or might in the future?

2. Do I feel tired/ sleepy tired?

3. How mentally awake do I feel?

4. How nervous or anxious do I feel?

5. Do I keep looking at my clock?

6. Am I focusing on how long I have been awake?

7. Am I worrying about work or other responsibilities?

8. Am I focusing on my pain once I notice it?

9. Am I feeling annoyed/ frustrated about something?

10. Am I considering how light/dark the room is?

11. Why can't I stop my mind from racing?

12. Am I thinking too much about ways I can get to sleep?

13. Am I thinking about the things I have to get done?

14. Am I focusing on noises I hear?

15. Am I thinking about the effects of not sleeping well?

16. Am I worrying about being awake all night?

17. Is the problem that I am over thinking things too much?

18. Am I focusing on how bad I am at sleeping?

19. Am I thinking about things in the past?

20. Am I concentrating too much on things to do to

   help me sleep?

12 steps to put the mind at rest

'Put the Day to Rest.'
The aim is to put the day to bed, along with all your plans for the next day, long before bedtime, so that when bed comes you can get to sleep. These 12 steps which can be carried out in about 20 minutes can help you manage your thoughts which you would usually take to bed and analyse!

1. Every early evening for example 8.00 pm, if possible set aside 20 minutes.
2. Sit somewhere quietly were you won't be disturbed.
3. Get out your journal or notebook and a pen.
4. Think about what sort of day it has been, what has happened during the day, how events have gone, and how you feel about the kind of day it has been.
5. Put them to rest by writing down the main points of your day in your journal or notebook. Remember to write down both what you feel good about and also what has troubled you.
6. In your journal or notebook, write yourself a 'to do list'. Be sure to include any steps that you can take to tie up any loose ends or unfinished business.
7. Spend some time considering tomorrow, what are your plans for tomorrow? Think about all the things that may cause you concern, but also think about things you are looking forward to, and write them down in your journal or notebook.
8. You may find it useful to get a diary and write your schedule down in there, or you can check things you have scheduled are in your diary

9. If there is anything you aren't sure of, make a note of it in your diary, journal or notebook. Importantly schedule a time the next day when you are going to find out the answers!
10. Use this allocated 20 minutes to leave you feeling more in control of today and prepared for tomorrow.
11. Just before bed, remind yourself that you have dealt with anything from that day.
12. Keep your journal or notebook by your bed so if you think of new things while in bed, just jot them down and deal with them tomorrow morning.

It's important to remember what you have already learned and use the information to evaluate your thoughts and attributes. As we have said earlier in this book, your attitude towards sleep and sleeplessness is so important.

Block out those trivial thoughts

This technique works best with trivial information that just comes to mind, rather than more serious problems. Thought-blocking works by stopping other thoughts from getting in. When interrupting thoughts come to you in the middle of the night, start thought-blocking immediately before you are wide awake.

How to stop those thoughts:
1. Close your eyes and repeat the word 'the' slowly and calmly every 2 seconds in your head
2. 'Mouth' the word rather than saying it out loud.
3. Try to continue this for about 5 minutes (If you can).

The word 'the' is meaningless and has no emotional effect. By repeating this word, it stops other thoughts getting into your mind, hence the term, thought-blocking.

Relaxation and Self hypnosis
In earlier chapters we have discussed the benefits of relaxation and talked about progressive muscular relaxation and self-hypnosis. To recap, relaxation is a good way to relax the mind and body. It is a good distraction technique which helps to focus your mind away from intrusive and worrying thoughts. Relaxation exercises can give you more of a sense of being in control – of your breathing, your muscles and your mind. Remember for relaxation and/or self-hypnosis, it has to be practiced regularly to be most effective.

Are you trying too hard to sleep?
"Sleep is like a cat: it only comes to you if you ignore it"
You cannot force yourself to sleep; the harder you try the less successful you are which leads to frustration, irritability and keeps you awake. These frustrations often lead to us exaggerating our emotions and thoughts about not being able to sleep for example "I'm the only person awake now". Sometimes, just going with the insomnia helps, as does a sense of humour. Accept that you can't sleep. Try to challenge your thoughts – realistically are you the only one in the world who isn't asleep? Maybe reframe your thoughts as discussed earlier, and see that being awake isn't such a bad thing as it provides opportunities for you to do things that you enjoy. Letting sleep strengthen and develop again naturally will take you closer to your goal of being a good sleeper.

People with insomnia strive to control their sleep. However, sleep is an involuntary physiological process, which cannot be placed under full voluntary control. Therefore, direct, voluntary attempts to control sleep may actually increase insomnia.

Alternatively use a paradoxical method, by that I mean completely give up trying to sleep. The classic example of this that is well quoted is that if you are told not to think about a pink elephant, you will do!

Change your goal, give up any effort to fall asleep, just lie peacefully in your bed with your eyes open and don't worry about just lying there not being able to sleep.

When your eyelids feel heavy and want to close, say to yourself that you are going to stay awake for just a little bit longer; but don't force yourself to stay awake.

What else is keeping you awake?

Are you paying too much attention to your sleep or lack or it? The techniques that have already been mentioned will help to reduce attention on sleep - Putting the day to rest, having a pre-bedtime routine, relaxation and imagery, thought-stopping and sleep-scheduling.

Are you clock watching? Often people with insomnia use the time as a performance indicator as well as using the clock to tell the time. This is part of the self-monitoring tendency that heightens arousal in bed and usually leads to negative self- evaluation. Therefore, your awareness of time often gets linked to an automatic and dysfunctional thought, creating a negative evaluation of one's self. Turn the clock around so you can't see the clock face, to avoid noticing the time every few minutes which seems like an hour!

Chapter 13

KEEPING IT GOING!

Firstly, let's congratulate yourself on getting this far with this book, I'm assuming that you have started to notice a positive change in your sleep patterns. Remember developing a good sleep pattern may take a number of weeks to establish and you need to be prepared for this. Although this book offers guidance towards your progress there is a lot you can do on your own. Implementing the instructions contained within these chapters is the hardest part, however in order to become a good sleeper it is important to do all of them! DO NOT PICK AND CHOOSE – follow the whole process.

So let's briefly recap the previous chapters:

The 'nuts and bolts'
- You need to think of insomnia as a bad habit that can be got rid of.

- Keep filling in your sleep diary for at least six weeks.
- You need to stick to the routines you develop until your sleep improves.
- In consultation with your GP, consider gradually reducing any sleeping pills that you take.
- As far as possible get a comfortable bed and mattress that suits you.
- Using your sleep diaries, work out your sleep schedule. Look at your average length of time asleep, the time you plan to get up in the morning, and threshold time for considering going to bed.
- Your threshold time is calculated by subtracting the average duration of your sleep at present from your time to get up in the morning.
- Follow your planned sleep schedule every night.
- Only make adjustments to your sleep schedule, once the amount of time you are asleep in bed reaches 90 percent.
- Only increase by a maximum rate of 15 minutes per week

Pre bedtime do's and don'ts

- If possible try to add some light exercise into your day, preferably in the late afternoon or early evening.
- Reduce the amount of coffee or tea that you drink, perhaps you could try de-caffeinated drinks.
- Reduce your smoking in the evening and try not to smoke if you wake during the night.
- Do not drink alcohol to help your sleep – it usually disrupts sleep as often you will have to get up to go to the bathroom.

- Do not sleep or nap in the armchair during the day. Keep sleep for bedtime and only sleep in bed.
- Make sure your bed and bedroom are comfortable – not too cold, warm, noisy or bright. The room should be well aired and the alarm clock turned towards the wall.
- Put the day to rest long before bedtime. Think it through, tie up 'loose ends' in your mind and plan ahead. Use your journal or notebook to write things down.
- Wind down during the evening and stick to your routine.
- Have a plan and make arrangements for waking during the night, such as leaving out some of your favourite 'help sleep' things such as CDs or colouring books, if possible make sure the heating is on low so you don't get too cold.

Do's and don'ts while in bed!
- Only go to bed when sleepy-tired and this must be after your threshold time. Being sleepy-tired will make you fall asleep more quickly and help you sleep through the night.
- The bedroom is only for sleeping. Do not read, watch TV, speak on the telephone, eat, drink, etc. in bed.
- Turn out the light as soon as you are in bed and lay your head on the pillow as you intend to go to sleep.
- Remember relaxation exercises or self-hypnosis should be practiced regularly to be effective.
- Don't try too hard to sleep; either adopt a more carefree attitude to being awake, perhaps accepting

that even if you aren't sleeping you are still resting. Alternatively try to keep your eyes open and try gently to resist sleep.

○ Have your alarm set to get up at the same time every day, seven days a week, and make sure you do get up at this time.

Tips for if you can't sleep or wake during the night

○ If you are not asleep within 15 minutes of going to bed, get up and go into a different room.

○ If you wake up in the middle of the night and can't get back to sleep within 15 minutes, get up, go into another room and do something.

○ If your pain always wakes you at the same time each night, set your alarm, 30 minutes earlier than you would normally wake and have your painkillers, this will help you feel that your sleep is less broken.

○ Try to avoid getting frustrated, angry or upset if you can't sleep or you wake up. Remember sleep problems are common!

○ Consider your negative and unhelpful thoughts about your sleep and/or pain and challenge them to prevent them taking over your thoughts, as we discussed in chapter eight.

○ Once sleepy-tired, go back to bed again. Turn out your light and practise self-hypnosis or some form of relaxation.

○ If your unhelpful thoughts persist, try to block them out by repeating the word 'the' to yourself every 2 seconds. Try to keep this up for 5 minutes at a time.

○ In your notebook or journal kept by your bed, write

down any negative or unhelpful thoughts and deal with them in the morning.

- **If after 15 minutes you are still not asleep, then get up and repeat the above steps as many times as you need to.**

Over to you - Let's review how far you have come . . .

○ What have I achieved?

○ What have I not achieved?

○ Which chapters of this book *are not* relevant to

me?

Final words

SLEEPING WITH PAIN IS POSSIBLE

Remember it will be useful to read this book or revisit chapters on a regular basis until you are happy with your sleep pattern. Relapses will occur and that's OK, just get back on track straight away.

This book is not intended to be a substitute for medical advice or treatment but to work alongside it. If you have a medical condition you should consult your GP or a qualified therapist.

If you follow the instructions set out in this book, you too will be able to fall asleep more quickly and sleep for longer periods of time throughout the night. This book has been based on a programme I use with patients and many of them have made big improvements. I would like to thank my patients over the years who have evaluated this programme frequently to enable me to improve it. Now it is in book format here, I hope it will help all of you with pain and problems sleeping who do not have access to a specialist pain clinic.

I would like to end this book by wishing you all the best for many nights sleeping successfully despite your pain!

Dr Sue Peacock

For more about chronic pain go to my website www.apaininthemind.co.uk and log on for lots of extra material using the password sandp124

Appendix

Who has insomnia?

Studies estimate that between a quarter and one-third of American and European adults experience some insomnia each year, with between 10 percent and 20 percent of them suffering severe sleeplessness.

In spite of this widespread problem, however, only about 30 percent of adults who visit their doctor ever discuss sleep problems and doctors seem rarely to ask patients about their sleep habits or problems.

The strongest risk factors for insomnia are psychiatric problems, particularly depression, and physical complaints, such as headaches and chronic pain that have no identifiable cause (called somatic symptoms). About 90 percent of people with depression have insomnia.

In addition, insomnia and depression often coincide with somatic symptoms, particularly chronic pain. In fact, insomnia worsens chronic pain even in people who are not depressed. Headaches that occur during the night or early in the morning may actually be caused by sleep disorders. In one study, patients who had these complaints were treated for the sleep disorder only, and over 65 percent reported that their headaches were cured. Overall, insomnia is more common in women than men, although men are not immune from insomnia. Sleep efficiency deteriorates equally in men and women as they get older.

One major study suggested that as men go from age 16 to 50, they lose about 80 percent of their deep sleep. During that period, light sleep increases and REM sleep remains unchanged. (The study did not use women as subjects, and there is some evidence to suggest they are not as affected.) After age 44 REM and total sleep diminish and awakenings increase.

Younger adult women suffer from insomnia because of both cultural and biological factors. As we've already examined, a number of hormonal events can disturb sleep, including premenstrual syndrome, menstruation, pregnancy, and menopause. All these conditions are natural, and in most cases the wakefulness associated with them is temporary and can be improved with sleep hygiene and time.

After childbirth, most women develop a high sensitivity to the sounds of their children, which causes them to wake easily. Women who have had children sleep less efficiently than women who have not had children. It is possible that many women never unlearn this sensitivity and continue to wake easily long after the children have grown.

After menopause women are susceptible to the same environmental and biological causes of insomnia as men are. Older women who are not bothered by sleeplessness tend to have longer and better sleep than non-insomniac men their own age.

Other groups of individuals who are likely to suffer from insomnia include those who travel frequently – especially when crossing time zones, those with post-traumatic stress syndrome, and individuals with brain injuries.

So, we have spent time discovering causes of insomnia other than your chronic pain, as most likely you will also be experiencing some of the other reasons for insomnia in addition to your chronic pain

sleeping with pain

Index

sleeping with pain

sleeping with pain

Printed in Great Britain
by Amazon